Guide

1.Introduction

To conquer a woman, it is essential to be yourself and show authenticity in everything you do. Women are attracted to self-assured, genuine, and authentic men, so it is important that you show your true personality and not try to be someone else just to impress her.

First of all, it is important to understand that a woman cannot be won over with clichéd phrases or fake attitudes. Sincerity is the key to winning a woman's heart, so try to always be honest and transparent with her. Show interest in what she says, listen carefully, and make her understand that your intentions are sincere.

Furthermore, it is important to be self-assured and have confidence in your abilities. Women are attracted to men who know how to value themselves and who are not afraid to show their weaknesses. Show confidence in yourself

Techniques to win over a woman

How to Win a Woman

Telma Sheller

A. Ludder

and your abilities, but do not fall into arrogance or presumption. Be humble and respectful towards the woman you want to conquer.

Moreover, it is essential to be authentic and show your personality genuinely. Do not try to be someone else, but let your true self shine through and allow the woman to get to know you for who you truly are. Show your interests, passions, and ambitions, in order to create an authentic and sincere connection.

It is also important to pay attention to details and demonstrate care and attention towards the woman you want to conquer. Small kind gestures, such as sending a message to see how she is doing or bringing her a small gift, can make a difference and show her how much you care about her.

Finally, it is crucial to be patient and respect the woman's timeline. Do not try to rush things, but let the relationship develop naturally and spontaneously. Show that you are available and interested, but respect her pace and needs.

To conquer a woman, it is essential to be yourself, authentic, and sincere. Show confidence in yourself, care and attention towards her, and let your authentic personality shine through. With the right mix of sincerity, confidence, and attention, you will be able to win over the heart of the woman you desire.

2. Show genuine interest in her interests and passions

When it comes to winning over a woman, showing genuine interest in her interests and passions is crucial. Women are attracted to men who demonstrate a desire to understand what makes them happy and to share their passions. Showing genuine interest will not only help create a deeper connection but will also demonstrate that you are an empathetic and caring person.

First and foremost, it's important to understand what it truly means to show genuine interest in a woman. It's not simply about listening to what she says and responding with generic phrases. It means truly taking the time to understand what she is passionate about and actively committing to supporting her in achieving her dreams and goals.

When you meet a woman you like, take the time to discover what her passions and interests are. It could be a hobby, a career, a project she's working on, or simply something that brings her joy. Ask her to tell you about herself and listen carefully to what she has to say. Ask thoughtful questions and show sincerity in your interest.

Once you have identified the passions of the woman you are interested in, look for ways to support and encourage her. You could offer your help or support in a project she's working on. Showing that you are willing to set aside your time and energy to help her achieve her dreams will be a sign of true interest and devotion.

Furthermore, actively participate in her passions and interests. If the woman you like is passionate about art, for example, you could accompany her to an art exhibition or gift her a book about an artist she loves. Showing that you are willing to share her passions and open yourself up to new experiences will help strengthen the bond between you.

Showing genuine interest in a woman's passions also means being empathetic and understanding. If the woman you like is facing challenges or difficult moments related to her passion, show her your support and understanding. Be there for her and offer your support so she feels heard and supported.

Lastly, it's important to be authentic in showing genuine interest. Do not pretend to be interested in a woman's passions just to win her over. Be sincere in your approach and be open in sharing your emotions and interests. Sincerity and authenticity are crucial in building a strong and lasting bond with a woman. Showing genuine interest in a woman's passions and interests is a fundamental step in winning her over. Being empathetic, understanding, and present in her life will make her feel loved and supported. Being open to sharing the passions of the woman you like will help strengthen the bond between you and create a deep and meaningful relationship.

3.Listen carefully and ask meaningful questions

Listening carefully and asking meaningful questions is crucial to winning over a woman. Often, men think they need to talk a lot about themselves to impress a woman, but the reality is that being a good listener is what truly makes a difference. In this article, we will explore the importance of listening and asking meaningful questions, and provide you with some tips on how to do so to win a woman's heart.

The art of active listening

Listening carefully is an art that requires practice and dedication. Many people tend to be distant during a conversation, thinking about what to say next rather than focusing on what the other person is saying. This not only leads to ineffective communication but also makes the other person feel like they are not truly interested in what they are saying.

To be a good listener, you must be present in the moment and focus on what the other person is communicating. Look them in the eyes, pay attention to their gestures and tone of voice. Show genuine interest in what they are saying and ask questions to delve deeper into their thoughts and feelings. This will not only make them feel appreciated but also allow you to get to know them better and build a stronger connection.

Asking meaningful questions

Asking questions is about trying to understand what the other person is communicating. This shows that you are interested in her and want to get to know her better. However, not all questions are equal. It is important to ask meaningful questions that allow the woman to express her thoughts and feelings in depth.

Avoid trivial questions like "how are you?" or "what do you do for a living?". Instead, try to ask questions that stimulate the conversation and allow the woman to express herself. For example, you could ask her what makes her smile, what her dream is, or what is most important to her in life. This will make her feel special and give her the opportunity to share her passions and values with you.

Tips for listening carefully and asking meaningful questions

To become an active listener and ask meaningful questions, follow these tips:

1. Put aside your distractions and focus on the other person. Eliminate distractions, such as your phone or external interruptions, and maintain eye contact to show interest.

2. Ask open-ended questions that allow the other person to express themselves freely. Avoid yes/no questions and try to ask questions that begin with "how", "what", or "why".

3. Listen with empathy and show understanding towards the other person's feelings and opinions. Avoid interrupting or judging them while they speak.

4. Repeat what they have said to show that you have listened carefully. For example, you could say "So you mean that..." or "It seems

like you said that...".

5. Show genuine interest in what they are saying and ask questions to deepen their perspective. Try to understand what motivates them and what makes them happy.

Listening carefully and asking meaningful questions is essential to winning over a woman. Being a good listener will allow you to create a deeper bond and get to know her better. Remember to put aside your distractions, show empathy, and ask questions that stimulate the conversation. Follow the tips provided in this article and you will be on your way to winning a woman's heart.

4. Give sincere and specific compliments

To win over a woman, it's not enough to just give generic and cliché compliments, but it's important to be sincere and specific to make her understand how much you truly value and appreciate her. The art of giving compliments is a skill that can make a difference in courtship and in creating a deep connection with the person you're interested in. In this article, we will give you some tips on how to give sincere and specific compliments to win over a woman.

First and foremost, it's crucial that the compliments are genuine and spontaneous. Women are very intuitive and can tell when someone is trying to flatter them just to get something in return. So, before giving a compliment, make sure it's authentic and truly reflects what you think of her.

An effective way to give a sincere and specific compliment is to notice the unique qualities of the person you're interested in. For example, you could say: "I really like your listening skills, it makes me feel truly heard and understood by you." In this way, you're showing appreciation for a specific characteristic of her personality that makes her special in your eyes.

Another important tip is to be specific in the compliments you give. Avoid being vague or generic, but instead, try to be precise in describing what you like about her. Instead of simply saying "You're beautiful," you could say: "I love how your eyes light up when you smile, it's really contagious." By doing this, you're showing that you've noticed something specific that has impressed and attracted you.

Furthermore, it's important to be creative in the compliments you give. Avoid the usual clichés and try to be original and unique in your praises. For example, instead of saying

"You're sweet," you could say: "I admire how you take care of the people around you, it shows how caring and selfless you are." This kind of personalized and original compliment will surely leave a positive impression in the mind of the woman you're interested in.

Lastly, never forget to make the person feel special and unique through your compliments. Show sincerely how much you care about her and how much you appreciate her qualities and traits. A well-made compliment can make a difference in creating an emotional and deep bond with the person you want to win over.

Giving sincere and specific compliments is a skill that can help you win over a woman in an authentic and meaningful way. Remember to be sincere, specific, creative, and make her feel special through your praises. With a bit of attention and sensitivity, you will surely be able to win the heart of the woman you desire.

5. Smile and maintain eye contact

Smiling and maintaining eye contact are two fundamental skills for establishing a connection with a woman and winning her over. These two gestures communicate confidence, openness, and interest, key elements for creating an emotional and empathetic bond with the person you are speaking to. In this article, we will delve into the importance of smiling and eye contact in seduction, providing practical tips on how to use these techniques effectively to attract and conquer a woman.

A smile is a powerful weapon in seduction. A genuine and sincere smile can convey sympathy, kindness, and positivity, making the person feel welcomed and appreciated. When you smile at a woman, you show her your best side, the one that makes her feel special and desired. A smile is also contagious: if you show a positive and cheerful attitude, the woman in front of you is likely to respond with a smile and be attracted to you.

But be careful: the smile must be authentic, otherwise you risk appearing fake and unconvincing. To have a natural and charming smile, you should think of something pleasant or funny, so that positive emotions are reflected on your face. Also, try to maintain a relaxed and unforced expression, avoiding stiffening your mouth or showing your teeth excessively. A spontaneous and sincere smile is much more attractive than one that is contrived.

Once you have learned to smile convincingly, it's time to focus on eye contact. Eye contact is an extremely powerful form of non-verbal communication, capable of conveying deep and emotional messages without saying a word. When you look a woman in the eyes, you show her your interest and attention, creating a direct and intense emotional bond.

However, eye contact can be a double-edged sword: if you stare too intensely or invasively, you risk making the other person uncomfortable and losing their interest. It is important to strike a balance between looking into someone's eyes and giving moments of pause, so as not to appear too insistent or invasive. Try alternating direct gazes with quick glances at other parts of the person's face or body, in order not to discomfort the woman.

Furthermore, it is important to be able to interpret the signals that a woman sends you through eye contact. If you notice that her pupils dilate when she looks at you, it is a sign of attraction and interest in you. Likewise, if she lowers her gaze and then quickly raises it, it could be a sign of shyness or embarrassment, but also desire and fascination. Learn to read the non-verbal signals that a woman sends you through eye contact, so as to adapt your behavior and respond to her emotions and feelings.

Finally, it is important to remember that smiling and maintaining eye contact are just two of the many seduction techniques that you can use to win over a woman. In addition to these skills, it is crucial to show kindness, gallantry, interest, and self-confidence, in order to make a good impression and arouse the interest of the person you are talking to. Remember that the key to winning over a woman is to be authentic, sincere, and respectful, showing your best side and making her feel special and desired.

Smiling and maintaining eye contact are two powerful gestures that can help you conquer a woman and establish a deep emotional bond with her. Learn to use these techniques effectively and naturally, showing your best side and highlighting your personal charm. With a sincere smile and a direct and intense gaze, you can attract and conquer the woman of your dreams, creating an emotional and empathetic bond that can last over time.

6. Show kindness and chivalry

Kindness and chivalry are two characteristics that never go out of style when it comes to winning a woman's heart. The ability to be kind and chivalrous not only makes a woman feel appreciated and loved, but also shows the respect and attention you have towards her. In this article, we will explore how to show kindness and chivalry in different situations to win a woman's heart.

Kindness is a quality that costs nothing but can make a difference when it comes to getting a woman's attention. Being kind means being caring, respectful, and polite, but also being able to listen and show empathy. Showing kindness can manifest in many different ways, such as holding the door open, offering help when needed, saying thank you and sorry when necessary, or simply being there when a woman needs comfort.

Chivalry, on the other hand, is an art that can make a woman feel like a princess and demonstrate your interest and respect towards her. Being chivalrous means being courteous, generous, and caring, but also knowing how to make romantic and thoughtful gestures to win her over. Chivalry can manifest in many ways, such as opening the car door, pulling out a chair for her to sit, offering your jacket when it's cold, or taking care of her with sweet and caring gestures.

When it comes to showing kindness and chivalry to win a woman over, it's important to do so sincerely and authentically, without any forced or false intentions. Women are able to perceive when a gesture is genuine and when it's just a tactic to get something in return. Showing kindness and chivalry should be a true way of life, a characteristic that is part of your personality and way of being.

One of the first rules for being kind and chivalrous to a woman is to always be respectful and polite. Never use vulgar or offensive language, never raise your voice or have abrupt attitudes. Education and respect are the basis of any healthy and lasting relationship, and are essential for winning a woman over. Being kind and chivalrous doesn't mean being weak or submissive, but on the contrary, it shows strength, security, and maturity.

Being kind and chivalrous to a woman also means being able to listen and show empathy towards her. Women love to feel heard and understood, and appreciate when someone is willing to listen to and understand their emotions and needs. Being a good listener is a fundamental skill to win a woman's heart, as it shows attention and interest towards her.

In addition to being kind and chivalrous with words, it's also important to demonstrate it through actions. Small acts of kindness and chivalry can make a difference when it comes to winning a woman over. For example, bringing her a bouquet of flowers or a box of chocolates, preparing a romantic candlelit dinner, giving her a book she likes, or simply giving her a hug when she needs it. Kind and chivalrous gestures can make a woman feel special and loved, and demonstrate your interest towards her.

Another important rule for being kind and chivalrous to a woman is to be patient. Winning a woman's heart is not something that can be done overnight, but takes time, commitment, and dedication. Being patient means showing understanding and respect for the woman's timeframe, listening to her and understanding her needs and desires, and being ready to support and stand by her in the decisions she makes. Patience is a virtue that deserves to be cultivated when it comes to winning a woman's heart.

Lastly, to win a woman over, it is essential to be authentic and genuine. Being kind and chivalrous does not mean pretending to be someone you're not, but being yourself and showing who you truly are. Women love sincerity and authenticity, and appreciate when someone is willing to be themselves without masks or filters. Being authentic and genuine is a quality that can make a difference when it comes to winning a woman's heart, as it shows trust and transparency towards the other person.

Showing kindness and chivalry is an effective way to win a woman's heart and make her feel special and loved. Being kind and chivalrous means being caring, respectful, polite, and being able to listen and show empathy towards the woman. Showing kindness and chivalry sincerely and authentically, with gestures and words, with patience and understanding, can make a difference when it comes to winning a woman's heart.

Remember, kindness and chivalry are the keys to open a woman's heart and win it forever.

7.Show confidence in yourself

In a romantic relationship, self-confidence plays a crucial role in ensuring the success of the relationship. In particular, when it comes to wooing a woman, self-assurance is as important as it is attractive. In fact, a person who demonstrates self-confidence exudes positive energy and a capacity to tackle life's challenges with determination and courage.

Self-confidence is a characteristic that can be developed and strengthened over time through self-esteem, self-awareness, and the ability to manage emotions in a balanced way. It is important to understand that self-confidence does not mean being arrogant or presumptuous, but rather being aware of one's qualities and strengths, while also accepting one's flaws and constantly working to improve.

To win over a woman, it is crucial to show confidence in oneself and one's abilities, demonstrating determination and clear goals in life. A person who knows what they want and puts effort into pursuing their goals is much more attractive in the eyes of the opposite sex. Self-confidence also manifests in the ability to communicate clearly and effectively, expressing one's opinions and feelings with security and respect.

Another important key to showing self-confidence in wooing a woman is the ability to make decisions independently and assertively, without being too influenced by others' opinions. Showing confidence in one's choices and behavior is an effective way to gain respect and admiration from the woman one desires to conquer.

To increase self-confidence, it is important to work on one's self-esteem and self-acceptance, learning to appreciate one's qualities and value one's peculiarities. Taking care of one's physical appearance and health can also help one feel more confident and project a better image of oneself to others.

Moreover, it is important to face one's limits and fears with courage and determination, seeking to overcome the obstacles and challenges that life presents. Showing the ability to tackle difficulties with resolve is a sign of self-confidence that will not go unnoticed by the woman one desires to conquer.

Finally, it is important to remember that self-confidence is a continuous process of personal growth and self-improvement. It is not a one-time goal to achieve, but a journey that requires constant commitment and dedication. Maintaining high self-confidence requires effort and perseverance, but the results that can be achieved are definitely worth every endeavor.

Showing confidence in oneself in wooing a woman is a key element in ensuring the success of a romantic relationship. Self-esteem, self-awareness, and the ability to manage emotions are fundamental aspects to cultivate in order to appear self-assured and attractive to the desired woman. Constantly working on one's self-confidence is a valuable investment that will certainly bring benefits in personal life and interpersonal relationships.

8.Maintain excellent personal hygiene

Dressing appropriately and neatly is a fundamental aspect of winning over a woman. Clothing speaks volumes about us and our personality, so it is important to pay attention to every detail to make a good impression. In this article, we will explore together what are the most suitable clothing items to conquer a woman and how to pair them best.

First of all, it is important to understand the context in which you find yourself and the type of woman you want to conquer. If it is a formal meeting, such as an elegant dinner or an important appointment, it is essential to wear an outfit appropriate for the situation. A stylish suit, composed of a coordinated jacket and pants, is always a winning choice. You can opt for a classic black or dark blue suit, paired with a white shirt and a matching tie. This look is perfect for conveying confidence and sophistication.

If it is a more informal date, such as a drink at the bar or a city stroll, you can choose a more casual yet well-groomed outfit. A pair of dark jeans paired with a checked shirt or an elegant t-shirt is an ideal choice. You can complete the look with a leather jacket or a blazer, for an extra touch of class. The important thing is to always maintain a balance between elegance and comfort, to avoid looking too formal or too sloppy.

An important detail not to overlook is attention to detail. A good cologne, a well-groomed beard, and orderly hair are elements that can make a difference and make the look even more appealing. It is also important to pay attention to the choice of accessories, which can complete the look and add a touch of personality. A high-quality belt, an elegant watch, or a coordinated pocket square are small details that can make a difference.

The choice of colors is another aspect to consider. Neutral tones like black, blue, and gray are always a safe choice because they are elegant and easy to match. However, do not be afraid to dare with brighter colors, which can add a touch of originality and personality to the look. It is important, however, not to overdo it and maintain a balance between the different colors, avoiding too obvious contrasts that could be excessive.

Finally, it is crucial to feel comfortable in the chosen clothing. Confidence and self-esteem are as attractive as a well-tailored suit, so it is important to feel good in what you wear. If you feel comfortable and confident, you will automatically transmit a positive energy that will be appreciated by the woman you want to conquer.

Dressing appropriately and neatly is a fundamental step in winning over a woman. Paying attention to every detail, from the choice of clothing to the care of the details, is a sign of respect and attention that will not go unnoticed. With a well-groomed and stylish look, combined with a good dose of confidence and self-esteem, we will be ready to win over the heart of our ideal woman.

9.Dress appropriately and neatly

Dressing appropriately and neatly is a fundamental aspect of winning over a woman. Clothing speaks volumes about us and our personality, so it is important to pay attention to every detail to make a good impression. In this article, we will explore together which clothing items are most suitable for winning over a woman and how to pair them effectively.

First and foremost, it is important to understand the context in which you find yourself and the type of woman you wish to win over. If it is a formal meeting, such as an elegant dinner or an important date, it is crucial to wear an outfit suitable for the occasion. A smart suit, consisting of a coordinated jacket and trousers, is always a winning choice. You can opt for a classic black or dark blue suit, paired with a white shirt and a coordinated tie. This look is perfect for conveying confidence and sophistication.

If it is a more casual date, such as a drink at a bar or a stroll in the city, you can choose a more casual yet still neat outfit. A pair of dark jeans paired with a plaid shirt or an elegant t-shirt is an ideal choice. You can complete the look with a leather jacket or a blazer, for an added touch of class. The key is to always maintain a balance between elegance and comfort, so as not to appear too formal or too sloppy.

An important detail not to overlook is attention to detail. A good cologne, a well-groomed beard, and tidy hair are elements that can make a difference and make the look even more attractive. It is also important to pay attention to the choice of accessories, which can complete the look and add a touch of personality. A high-quality belt, an elegant watch, or a coordinated pocket square are small details that can make a difference.

The choice of colors is another aspect to consider. Neutral tones such as black, blue, and gray are always a safe choice, as they are elegant and easy to match. However, do not be afraid to dare with brighter colors, which can add a touch of originality and personality to the look. It is important, however, not to overdo it and maintain a balance between different colors, avoiding too obvious contrasts that could be excessive.

Finally, it is crucial to feel comfortable in the clothing chosen. Confidence and self-esteem are as attractive as a well-tailored suit, so it is important to feel good in what you are wearing. If you feel comfortable and confident, you will automatically transmit a positive energy that will be appreciated by the woman you wish to win over. Dressing appropriately and neatly is a fundamental step in winning over a woman. Paying attention to every detail, from clothing choices to the care of details, is a sign of respect and attention that will not go unnoticed. With a well-groomed and elegant look, coupled with a good dose of confidence and self-esteem, we will be ready to win over the heart of our ideal woman.

10.Use humor to make her laugh

In recent years, humor has become increasingly important in seduction and courtship. A woman who laughs is a happy woman, and making her laugh is a sure way to win her over. But how can you be funny without seeming forced or ridiculous? In this article, we will explore different strategies and techniques to effectively and appropriately use humor to conquer a woman.

First of all, it is important to understand what kind of humor the woman you are trying to conquer likes. Some people prefer a sarcastic and cutting style, while others may appreciate a more gentle and good-natured style. Pay close attention to the woman's reactions to jokes and jokes to understand what makes her laugh the most.

One of the most effective techniques to make a woman laugh is the ability to use self-deprecation. Joking about oneself shows a certain amount of humility and self-awareness, two qualities highly appreciated by women. However, it is important not to overdo self-deprecation to avoid appearing insecure or lacking in confidence.

Another way to use humor to conquer a woman is to make jokes about current events or everyday life. A funny comment on a common situation or a news event can break the ice and generate a healthy laugh. However, it is important to be careful not to be too politically correct or offensive, especially at the beginning of a relationship.

Furthermore, it is important to be spontaneous and original in your jokes. Avoid reducing your repertoire to clichéd or already heard jokes, instead try to think of specific situations or details that can generate a genuine laugh. Originality is a trait highly appreciated by women, and using it in your humor can help you stand out from other suitors.

Another very effective technique to make a woman laugh is to use situational humor. Pay close attention to the situation you are in and try to pick out funny details or situations to exploit in your jokes. For example, if you are waiting for your order at a restaurant and the waitress brings you the wrong dish, you can make a light-hearted joke about the situation to make your companion laugh.

Finally, it is important not to overdo it with jokes or pranks. Even though making a woman laugh is a great way to win her over, it is important to be careful not to be too intrusive or insistent with jokes if they are not appreciated. Everyone has their own sense of humor, and it is important to respect the tastes and sensitivities of others.

Using humor to make a woman laugh is a great way to win her over. However, it is important to find the right balance between fun and respect, and to try to be original and spontaneous in your jokes. With a little

practice and attention, you will surely be able
to make your woman laugh and conquer her
with your humor.

11.Surprise her with romantic gestures

Surprising a woman with romantic gestures is a wonderful way to make her feel special and loved. It doesn't matter how long you have known each other or how long you have been together, showing your partner that you care about her and that you are committed to making her happy is always important. Romantic gestures can vary from small daily attentions to more elaborate surprises, but the important thing is that they are sincere and thoughtfully planned for her.

One of the simplest romantic gestures is sending sweet messages or leaving love notes in unexpected places, like her bag or her favorite book. A sweet message in the morning or before bedtime can make her feel loved and thought of even when you are not physically together. Even a small gift, like chocolate or a bouquet of flowers, for no reason can make her smile and appreciate your thoughtfulness.

Another idea to surprise her is to organize a romantic dinner at home or book a table at an elegant restaurant. You can cook together her favorite dish or order from a restaurant she loves and create an intimate atmosphere with candles and romantic music. You can also prepare a picnic in a park or by the seaside and spend time together away from everyday life.

If you want to make a more significant gesture, you can plan a romantic mini vacation or a weekend getaway. Plan a trip to a place she has been wanting to visit for a long time or book a hotel room in a nearby city to explore new places together and have new experiences. Even a simple bike ride or a sunset stroll can be romantic if it is meant to make her feel special.

A romantic gesture that never goes out of style is writing a hand-written love letter. Express your deepest feelings and tell her how important she is to you, without fear of showing your vulnerability. A personal and sincere love letter can move her and make her understand how much you truly love her.

If you want to surprise her in an original way, you can organize a themed night or create a romantic adventure game. You can organize a treasure hunt at home, with clues that will lead her to find a special gift, or prepare a puzzle that reveals a secret message when completed. The important thing is to put your creativity at the service of love and make her understand how much you are willing to do to make her happy.

Finally, never forget the importance of dedicating quality time to her. Listen carefully to what she has to say, support her in her passions and interests, and make her feel important and loved every day. Romantic gestures can be grand and spectacular, but it is the small gestures of daily love that make the

difference and keep the flame of passion and
love alive in your relationship.

Surprising a woman with romantic gestures is
a wonderful way to win her heart and make
her feel loved and appreciated. Be creative
and think of gestures that are special and
meaningful to her, show her how much you
care about her well-being, and dedicate
quality time together. With a little effort and a
lot of love, you can win her over and make her
fall in love more and more each day.

12.Plan original and meaningful dates

If you're tired of the same old movie or dinner dates, it's time to change tactics and plan original and meaningful dates. Get inspired by the following ideas to make your meetings even more special and memorable.

1. Sunset picnic

Nothing is more romantic than a picnic at sunset. Pack a basket with delicious sandwiches, cheeses, and fresh fruit and head to a nearby park or green area. Bring a blanket and enjoy the tranquility of the moment as the sun slowly sets on the horizon.

2. Visit to an antique market

If you love art and antiques, plan a visit to a flea market or antique fair. You could stroll among the stalls in search of unique and special items to add to your personal collection.

3. Mountain hike

If you love nature and adventure, a mountain hike could be the perfect date. Choose a scenic route and enjoy the breathtaking scenery as you walk hand in hand. Remember to bring water and a snack to recharge your energy during the journey.

4. Blindfold dinner

For a unique sensory experience, plan a blindfold dinner. Book a table at a restaurant that offers this particular experience and let your senses guide you as you taste different dishes without seeing what you are eating. This date will allow you to connect with yourself and with each other in a deep and meaningful way.

5. Cooking class

If you love to cook, why not take a cooking class together? You could learn to prepare new and tasty dishes under the guidance of an experienced chef and have fun experimenting in the kitchen. At the end of the class, you can enjoy your creations together and maybe recreate them at home for another special dinner.

6. Visit an art exhibition

If you are passionate about art, a visit to an exhibition could be a stimulating and meaningful date. You could admire works by famous artists or discover new talents in the world of contemporary art. Discuss what you see and compare your opinions to enrich your dialogue.

7. Volunteering

If you want to do something meaningful for others, why not dedicate some time to volunteering together? You could choose to volunteer for an association that helps those in need or animals in distress. Working together for a common cause will allow you to share a meaningful experience that will bring you even closer together.

8. Board game night

If you love board games, organize a night dedicated to games with friends. You could challenge each other to Monopoly, Trivial Pursuit, or a more strategic board game. Healthy competition will allow you to have fun together and create unforgettable memories.

9. Moonlit walk

There is nothing more romantic than a moonlit walk. Choose a quiet and romantic place, such as a deserted beach or a silent park, and enjoy the magic of the night together. Breathe in the fresh air, listen to the sounds of nature, and let the moonlight envelop you in a romantic atmosphere.

10. Dance lesson

If you want to heat up the atmosphere and have fun together, why not book a dance lesson? You could learn to dance salsa, tango, or swing and spend a fun and active evening. Dancing together will allow you to create a strong emotional bond and share moments of joy and complicity.

Planning original and meaningful dates is a way to strengthen the bond with your loved one and create unforgettable memories together. Choose from the ideas above or be inspired by your imagination to create a special date that reflects your interests and passions. The important thing is to spend quality time together and nurture your relationship authentically and genuinely.

13. Invite her out and show her that you are interested in spending time with her

When it comes to winning over a woman, it is important to show interest not only in her, but also in the time that could be spent together. Inviting her out is a fundamental step in demonstrating your interest and showing that you want to deepen your mutual understanding. In this article, we will explore different strategies and tips on how to invite a woman out and make it clear that you want to spend time together.

First and foremost, it is important to understand that every woman is different and therefore there is no magic formula to win them all over. It is essential to know her interests, preferences and try to adapt to them when deciding to invite her out. Showing attention and care towards the person you want to win over is a fundamental step in making her understand that you are genuinely interested in her.

When deciding to invite a woman out, it is important to do it with the right timing. You should not rush, but you should not wait too long either. Finding the right moment to ask to spend time together is essential to ensure that the proposal is accepted enthusiastically and not seen as an imposition or as a request that is too invasive.

It is also important to show sincerity and be clear about your intentions. If you truly want to spend time with a woman, it is important to say it openly and sincerely, without hiding your feelings or intentions. Transparency is crucial to creating a solid foundation on which to build a healthy and lasting relationship.

One way to invite a woman out and make it clear that you want to spend time with her is to plan a special date. This could mean organizing a romantic dinner, a night at the cinema, a walk in the park, or any other activity that is enjoyable for the person you want to win over. Showing interest in doing something special together is a way to demonstrate that you want to make the time spent together unique and significant.

It is also important to be kind, caring, and respectful towards the woman you want to win over. Education and respect are essential to make her understand that you are reliable and respectful individuals, and that you want to take the relationship you want to build with her seriously. Showing attention to detail, being thoughtful, and showing interest in her passions and interests are all ways to demonstrate your genuine interest.

Another strategy to invite a woman out and make it clear that you want to spend time with her is to show interest in her life and emotions. Asking her to share her experiences, dreams, and fears is a way to demonstrate that you are genuinely interested in getting to know her deeply and understanding who she truly is. Showing empathy and understanding towards the person you want to win over is essential to create a deep and meaningful bond.

Finally, it is important to show confidence in yourself and your abilities. Being self-assured and trusting in your ability to win over a woman is crucial to convey confidence and security to the person you want to conquer. Showing self-assurance, positivity, and determination is a way to make her understand that you are strong and optimistic individuals, ready to overcome any obstacle that may arise in the relationship.

In conclusion, inviting a woman out and showing that you want to spend time with her is a fundamental step in winning her over and creating a deep and meaningful relationship. Showing interest, care, kindness, and respect are essential to make her understand that you want to build something unique and special with her. Following the suggestions and strategies described in this article can help win over the heart of your loved one and create an authentic and lasting relationship.

14.Show assertive and decisive, but always respect her choices

Being assertive and decisive without overstepping the boundaries of respect and others' choices is a fundamental characteristic to genuinely and respectfully win over a woman. Women appreciate men who know what they want and are able to communicate it clearly and directly, but at the same time, are able to respect others' opinions and choices. In this article, we will explore how to show assertiveness and decisiveness without being intrusive or overbearing, to win a woman's heart in an authentic and sincere way.

First of all, it is important to understand that being assertive does not mean being aggressive or dominant. Being assertive means expressing one's opinions and desires clearly and directly, without forcing others to follow us or agree with us. It is important to be aware of one's own emotions and needs, and to be able to communicate them in a calm and composed way.

Furthermore, it is important to be decisive in one's actions and choices. Women appreciate men who are confident and know what they want from life. However, being decisive does not mean being rigid or inflexible, but being aware of one's priorities and goals and acting accordingly to achieve them.

To show assertiveness and decisiveness, it is important to work on oneself and on self-esteem. Being self-assured is essential to communicate one's opinions and desires clearly and directly. Engaging in activities that challenge us and allow us to develop a sense of self-efficacy can help us become more confident in ourselves and our abilities.

It is also important to be aware of one's emotions and learn to manage them in a healthy and balanced way. Women appreciate men who are able to express their emotions authentically and sincerely, without losing control of themselves. Learning to communicate empathetically and kindly, listening and respecting others' emotions, is essential to create a deep and lasting emotional bond with a woman.

When it comes to winning over a woman, it is important to show interest and attentiveness to her needs and desires. Listening to her attentively and showing empathy for her experiences and emotions can make the difference between a simple flirt and a meaningful and deep relationship. Showing interest in what the woman has to say and what makes her happy is essential to create an authentic and lasting bond.

However, it is important to remember that being assertive and decisive does not mean yielding to others' desires. It is essential to respect one's own opinions and choices, even if they may differ from those of the woman we are trying to win over. Showing assertiveness does not mean being overbearing or egocentric, but rather being able to express one's opinions and desires clearly and respectfully.

Furthermore, it is important to have confidence in one's abilities and value as individuals. Women appreciate men who are self-assured and who respect and value themselves for who they are. Being assertive and decisive also means being able to put oneself out there and show oneself for who they truly are, without masks or pretenses.

Lastly, it is important to be patient and respectful towards the woman you are trying to win over. Everyone has their own timing and needs, and it is important to respect them without trying to force the situation. Showing empathy and kindness, listening and understanding others' needs and desires, can make the difference between a superficial conquest and an authentic and meaningful relationship.

Being assertive and decisive is essential to win over a woman in an authentic and respectful way. Showing confidence in oneself and one's opinions, being decisive in one's actions and choices, being empathetic and kind towards others are qualities that can make the difference between a superficial conquest and a deep and lasting relationship. Remembering to always respect others' choices and to be patient and kind can help build a strong and deep bond with the woman of our dreams.

15.Show empathy and understanding when necessary

Showing empathy and understanding are essential qualities to win over a woman in an authentic and meaningful way. Showing a woman that you have the ability to understand and share her feelings and emotions can make the difference between a superficial relationship and a deep, authentic connection.

The ability to put yourself in someone else's shoes and understand their perspectives, needs, and desires is crucial for building a healthy and lasting relationship. Being empathetic means being able to listen carefully to what the woman has to say, without interrupting or judging her. Showing genuine interest in her thoughts and feelings, and demonstrating that you are available to support and understand her needs can make her feel secure and appreciated.

Understanding is another important quality to show when trying to win over a woman. Being able to understand her past experiences and fears will help you create a deeper bond with her. Showing that you are willing to make an effort to get to know her inner world and accept her imperfections will make you more attractive to her.

To show empathy and understanding when necessary, it is essential to be present and attentive during conversations with the woman you desire to conquer. Avoid distractions and focus on her, listening carefully to what she has to say and responding appropriately. Show interest in her interests, passions, and goals and try to understand what makes her happy or sad.

If the woman you desire to conquer is going through a difficult time or showing feelings of sadness, worry, or frustration, be open to sharing her emotions and offering your support. You may not necessarily try to solve her problems, but show her that you are there for her and that you can be a point of reference and comfort when she needs it.

Being empathetic and understanding also involves being able to communicate your feelings and thoughts openly and honestly. Do not be afraid to show vulnerability and express your emotions in order to create an atmosphere of mutual trust and authenticity. Sincerity and transparency are crucial for building an authentic and deep connection with the woman you desire to conquer.

Showing empathy and understanding when necessary is an effective way to demonstrate to the woman you are trying to conquer that you are an empathetic, compassionate partner who is interested in understanding and supporting her. These qualities are essential for creating a relationship based on trust, mutual understanding, and respect, and for building an authentic and meaningful connection that can last over time.

16.Be available and present when she needs you

When it comes to winning over a woman, one of the most important aspects is knowing how to be available and present when she needs you. Showing interest and attention towards the person you are interested in is crucial to creating an emotional bond and building a strong and lasting relationship. In this article, we will explore the importance of being present and available to win a woman's heart.

Being available does not mean being always available 24 hours day , but rather being willing to listen, support, and be present when the person you are interested in needs you. Being present means being physically and mentally present, valuing her needs, desires, and emotions.

When a woman realizes that you can be a constant and reliable presence in her life, she will be more likely to trust you and open up emotionally. Being available and present does not mean being clingy or intrusive, but rather demonstrating interest and attention in a balanced and sincere way.

Being available and present also means being empathetic and understanding towards the person you are interested in. Listening without judgment, showing empathy towards her feelings, and respecting her opinions are essential components for creating a deep and authentic emotional bond.

When a woman knows she can rely on you at any time, she will feel safe and protected, and will be more likely to open up and share her deepest thoughts and feelings with you. Being a constant reference point in a woman's life is an effective way to win her heart and build a meaningful and fulfilling relationship.

Being present when she needs you also means

being ready to support and assist the person you love in times of difficulty and crisis. Being available to offer comfort, emotional support, and practical solutions when the person you are interested in is going through a tough time is a sign of maturity and genuine interest in her well-being.

Showing empathy and understanding towards the challenges and problems that the person you love faces is an effective way to demonstrate your commitment and dedication to the relationship. Being present when she needs you is a way to show that you are willing to make an effort to ensure that your relationship thrives and grows over time.

Being available and present when she needs you also means being willing to compromise and put aside your own needs and desires to meet those of the person you love. Being willing to make concessions and prioritize the well-being and happiness of the person you are interested in is a sign of maturity and deep respect towards her.

Being available and present when she needs you also means being attentive to non-verbal signals and the needs of the person you love. Being able to read and interpret her facial expressions, body language, and emotions will allow you to better understand her needs and be a more empathetic and understanding partner.

Being present when she needs you does not mean doing everything alone, but rather being a collaborative and assertive partner who keeps up with the needs of the person you love. Being able to actively listen, communicate clearly, and respect the opinions and desires of the person you love are key skills to keep the flame of passion and love alive in your relationship.

Being present when she needs you is a way to show that you care about the person you love and are willing to make sacrifices for her well-being and happiness. Being a present and reliable partner is an effective way to win a woman's heart and build a strong and lasting relationship based on trust and mutual respect.

Being available and present when she needs you is essential to winning the heart of a woman and building a strong and fulfilling relationship. Showing interest, attention, and availability towards the person you are interested in is an effective way to create a deep and authentic emotional bond that can last over time. Be ready to support and assist the person you love in every moment and situation, and you will see that her heart will be yours forever.

17.Surprise her with small gifts specifically tailored for her

The relationship with a woman can be made even more special and intense through sweet gestures and attentions specifically tailored for her. Surprising her with small gifts that are personalized and reflect her passions and desires is a great way to show your love and attention towards her.

It is often thought that in order to impress a woman, one must spend large sums of money on expensive and luxurious gifts. However, it is often the simplest and most meaningful gestures that touch a woman's heart and make her feel truly special.

In this article, we will give you some tips on how to surprise your loved one with small gifts specifically tailored for her, to conquer her and make her feel loved and appreciated.

1. Listen to her desires and interests

In order to choose the perfect gift for your loved one, it is important to listen to her desires and interests. Observe what she enjoys doing in her free time, what are her hobbies and passions. For example, if she loves reading, you could gift her a book by an author she particularly loves or a book she has been wanting to read for a while.

If she is a creative person and enjoys art, you could consider gifting her materials for her hobby, like paints or a sketchbook to preserve her drawings. The important thing is to show her that you know her interests and that you care about what makes her happy.

2. Give experiences

Material gifts are often forgotten over time, while experiences lived together remain etched in memory forever. To conquer a woman, you could consider giving her an unforgettable experience, like a trip to a city she has been wanting to visit for a long time or a romantic dinner at an exclusive restaurant.

Experiences lived together strengthen the bond between two people and allow for the creation of unforgettable memories that will stay in the heart forever. Additionally, giving experiences is a way to show your loved one that you care about her happiness and that you desire to create special moments together with her.

3. Personalize the gifts

A way to make a gift even more special is to personalize it based on the tastes and preferences of your loved one. You could, for example, gift her a piece of jewelry with her name engraved or a unique and original design bag that reflects her personality.

Choosing handmade gifts can also be a great idea to show your commitment and attention towards your loved one. For example, you could create a photo album with your most meaningful photos together or a sweet treat made by you with your own hands.

4. Surprise her with unexpected gifts

To conquer a woman, it is important to know how to surprise her with unexpected gestures that make her feel special. For example, you could organize a surprise dinner at your home or rent a limousine to take her on a romantic ride around the city.

Even unexpected gifts, like a bouquet of flowers on a random day or an unexpected love letter, can make a difference and make your loved one feel loved and appreciated.

5. Listen to her needs and desires

To conquer a woman, it is important to show interest not only in her interests and passions, but also in her needs and desires. For example, if your loved one has been wanting a particular object for a long time, you could consider giving it to her to show her that you care about her aspirations and desires.

Giving something that can help her in her daily life, like a book that motivates her to achieve her goals or a useful accessory for her favorite sport activity, can show your loved one that you desire to support her and make her happy.

Conclusion

Surprising a woman with small gifts specifically tailored for her is a great way to show your love and attention towards her. In addition to giving material objects, it is important to think about gifts that are meaningful and reflect your loved one's personality and desires.

Listening to her interests, giving unforgettable experiences, personalizing gifts, surprising her with unexpected gestures, and taking care of her needs and desires are just some ways to conquer a woman and make her feel truly special.

Always remember that it is not the material value of the gift that makes a difference, but the care and attention you put into choosing something that is truly meaningful for your loved one. With sweet gestures and attentions specifically tailored for her, you will be able to conquer her and make her feel loved and appreciated like never before.

18. Demonstrate Your Commitment and Sincerity in Actions and Words

To win a woman's heart, it is crucial to demonstrate your commitment and sincerity through meaningful actions and words that truly reflect your feelings. Women are sensitive and attentive to details, so it is important to be genuine and authentic in showing your affection.

One of the first things to do to show your commitment and sincerity is to be consistently present in the life of the woman you wish to win over. Show interest in her passions, her interests, and her life in general. Be available to support her during difficult times and to celebrate joyful moments together.

It is also important to be respectful and courteous in both actions and words. Showing kindness and attention to the woman you want to win over is essential to let her understand how much you care about her and how far you are willing to go to make her happy.

Another way to demonstrate your commitment and sincerity is to be transparent and honest in your communications. Clearly express your feelings and intentions without hiding anything. Sincerity is fundamental for building a solid and lasting relationship, so it is important to be open and honest from the very beginning.

Additionally, demonstrating your commitment and sincerity through small attentions and affectionate gestures can make a difference. Giving flowers, writing sweet letters or messages, preparing a romantic dinner are just a few of the many possibilities to win a woman over and show her how important she is to you.

Being willing to listen and understand the needs and desires of the woman you want to win over is essential for building a healthy and balanced relationship. Showing empathy and understanding can make a difference in winning a woman's heart and making her feel truly loved and appreciated.

Finally, it is important to be consistent in your actions and words. Demonstrating your commitment and sincerity through consistent behavior over time is essential to show the woman you want to win over how serious and determined you are in your feelings.

To win a woman's heart, it is crucial to demonstrate your commitment and sincerity through meaningful actions and words that truly reflect your feelings. Being present, kind, transparent, affectionate, and empathetic are just some of the qualities that can help you

win a woman's heart and build a happy and
lasting relationship.

85

19. Do things together that she likes and that make her happy

A woman's happiness is one of the keys to winning her heart and keeping her happy and satisfied in a relationship. When it comes to doing things together that she likes and that make her happy, it is important to pay attention to her preferences and desires to ensure that you make choices that will make her happy.

In this article, we will explore some ideas and suggestions on what to do to win a woman and keep her happy, focusing on activities that you know she likes and that are important to her.

1. Listen and learn her preferences

One of the first things to do to win a woman and make her happy is to listen carefully to her preferences and desires. Ask her what her favorite activities are, what she likes to do in her free time, and what makes her happy. Once you understand her preferences, try to organize activities that align with her interests and make her happy.

2. Plan romantic dates

Women love romantic surprises and special dates, so plan some to make her feel loved and special. Plan a romantic dinner at home or in a restaurant, organize a day trip, or plan a night at the movies or the theater. Show her that you care about her and want to make every moment spent together special.

3. Give thoughtful gifts

Nothing makes a woman feel more loved and appreciated than a thoughtful gift specifically chosen for her. Try to understand her tastes and interests and give her something that you know she will appreciate. It could be a book by an author she loves, a designer item she has been wanting, or a day of relaxation at a spa. Show her that you are interested in her and care for her needs and desires.

4. Plan sports activities together

If your woman loves sports or physical activity, plan sports activities together to spend quality time together and have fun. You could go for a bike ride, a run in the park, or a yoga session together. The important thing is to find an activity that both of you enjoy and that allows you to strengthen your bond.

5. Cook for her

There is nothing more romantic than preparing a home-cooked dinner for your woman. Surprise her with a carefully prepared and lovingly cooked dinner, perhaps with her favorite dishes or with a gourmet dish that you know she will like. Light candles, play romantic music, and create an intimate and welcoming atmosphere that will make her feel loved and happy.

6. Support her in difficult times

One of the most important things to do to win a woman and keep her happy is to be by her side in difficult times. Show her your support and solidarity when she is going through moments of stress, worry, or sadness. Listen to her, comfort her, and let her know that you are there for her in every moment, both in happy and sad times.

7. Plan romantic getaways

Romantic getaways are a great way to spend quality time together and strengthen your bond. Plan a romantic getaway to a special place that you know she will appreciate, such as a tropical beach, an art city, or a luxury resort. Enjoy unforgettable moments together and create beautiful memories to share.

8. Participate in her favorite activities

To make her happy, it is important to participate in activities that she loves and that make her happy. If your woman loves shopping, watching movies, playing sports, or volunteering, join her and enjoy quality time together. Your participation in her favorite activities will show your interest in her and your desire to share special moments together.

9. Write her love letters

Women love to feel loved and appreciated, so write her love letters to express your feelings and emotions. Put into words everything you love about her, the special moments you have shared, and the emotions you feel when you are with her. Love letters are a romantic and sincere way to make her feel your love and dedication.

10. Dedicate time just for her

Lastly, to win her over and make her happy, it is important to dedicate quality time just for her. Plan romantic evenings, special days, or romantic weekends just for the two of you to strengthen your bond and create special moments to share. Show her that you are willing to invest time and energy in her and to make your relationship unique and special.

Doing things together that your woman loves and that make her happy is one of the secrets to winning her over and keeping her happy. Listen to her, fulfill her desires, surprise her with romantic gestures, and show her your love and support at all times. With a little dedication, attention, and care, you can win her heart and build a strong and happy relationship together.

20.Taking Care of Your Partner When She is Sick or Needs Help

Taking care of your partner when she is sick or needs help is a gesture that shows affection, care, and attention towards the loved one. Demonstrating support and presence during difficult times can strengthen the bond of the relationship. In this article, we will explore some tips on how to take care of her when she is sick or needs help, to win her heart and make her happy.

First of all, it is important to be empathetic and understanding towards your partner when she is in poor health. Let her express her emotions, listen to her actively, and show willingness to offer your help in any way possible. A caring and compassionate attitude, combined with concrete actions, can make a difference in comforting her and making her feel protected.

In case of illness, it is essential to ensure that your partner receives the necessary care to recover as quickly as possible. Accompanying her to the doctor, obtaining the prescribed medications, and assisting her with recommended therapies are gestures that demonstrate attention and concern for her well-being. Additionally, it is important to ensure that your partner follows a proper diet and gets enough rest to promote a speedy recovery.

During convalescence, it is crucial to spend time pampering her and making her stay at home more pleasant. Preparing nutritious and tasty meals, creating a comfortable and welcoming environment, and organizing relaxing activities can help her feel loved and supported. Paying attention to details and showing care in every gesture can make her feel special and appreciated.

Furthermore, it is important to be available to handle household chores and daily responsibilities to ease the workload of the sick partner. Cleaning the house, doing the shopping, taking care of household tasks, and managing any errands can allow her to rest and focus on her recovery. Demonstrating dedication and responsibility towards your partner can make her feel protected and loved.

In emergency situations or more serious cases, it is important to act promptly and calmly to ensure your partner's well-being. Staying calm, calling for help if necessary, and assisting her with professionalism and competence can be crucial in effectively handling critical situations. Showing determination and readiness in making important decisions can convey confidence and security to your partner in times of difficulty.

To win a woman's heart and make your partner happy, it is essential to demonstrate care and attention in moments of need and vulnerability. Taking care of her when she is sick or needs help is a gesture of love and respect that can strengthen the bond of the relationship. Showing empathy, understanding, and willingness to offer your support in a sincere and generous way can make her feel loved and appreciated.

Taking care of your partner when she is sick or needs help is an act of affection and care that can make a difference in the relationship. Showing attention to details, demonstrating dedication and responsibility, and offering your support in a sincere and generous way can help win a woman's heart and make her happy. Taking care of her when she needs it is a gesture of love and respect that can strengthen the bond of the relationship and make it stronger and more lasting.

21. Communicating openly and sincerely about your feelings and thoughts

Communicating openly and sincerely about one's feelings and thoughts is a fundamental aspect of building a healthy and lasting relationship with someone. In a romantic context, being able to openly express what one feels and thinks can make the difference between a superficial relationship and one that is deep and meaningful.

When it comes to winning over a woman, the ability to communicate openly and sincerely becomes even more important. Women are generally more empathetic and attuned to the emotions of others, so the ability to offer them a window into one's inner world can make them more likely to form a deeper emotional connection.

To communicate openly and sincerely with a woman, it is important to first be aware of one's own feelings and thoughts. Before sharing one's emotions with someone else, it is crucial to connect with oneself and understand what one truly feels. This means being honest with oneself and not being afraid to face uncomfortable or unpleasant emotions. Only once one is aware of their own feelings can they hope to effectively communicate them to others.

Once aware of their own feelings, it is important to find the right moment to communicate them to the woman one is trying to win over. Open and sincere communication requires a certain amount of vulnerability, so it is important to ensure that the person you are talking to is ready to receive your thoughts and feelings without judgment or harsh reactions.

When communicating with a woman, it is important to be authentic and sincere. People can tell when someone is not being genuine, and this can undermine the trust and sincerity of the relationship. To win over a woman with honesty and openness, it is important to be true to oneself and not be afraid to show one's true self.

To effectively communicate one's feelings and thoughts to a woman, it is important to listen carefully and show empathy. Communication is a two-way process, so it is important not only to express oneself but also to be able to listen and understand the other person. Showing empathy towards the woman demonstrates that you respect and understand her feelings and thoughts, creating a deeper emotional bond.

To win over a woman with open and sincere communication, it is also important to be respectful and kind. Kindness and respect are crucial for building a healthy and positive relationship with someone. Showing respect to the woman and treating her with kindness demonstrates that you pay attention to her needs and sensitivities, creating an atmosphere of trust and mutual sympathy.

Finally, to win over a woman with open and sincere communication, it is essential to be patient and consistent. Building a deep and meaningful relationship takes time and commitment, so it is important to be patient and consistent in communicating your feelings and thoughts. Honesty and openness are a solid foundation on which to build a lasting relationship, but it is important to consistently demonstrate them over time to strengthen the emotional bond with the woman you love.

22.Respect Her Space and Privacy Needs

When it comes to winning a woman's heart, there are many things you can do to make her feel loved, desired, and respected. Among these, one of the most important is certainly respecting her space and privacy needs. This means understanding that everyone needs a certain degree of intimacy and freedom, and it's essential to respect her choices and desires.

When getting to know a woman and wanting to win her over, it's important not to be intrusive and not to try to control her every move. Everyone has the right to maintain some privacy and to have moments for themselves, and it's important to respect this need when in a relationship.

One of the first things you can do to show respect for a woman's privacy is to ask for her consent before doing something that might invade her personal space. For example, if you want to enter her room or office, it's important to ask for permission before doing so. Additionally, it's important to respect her time and not try to impose your presence at every moment of the day.

Another important thing to do is to listen to and respect her boundaries. Everyone has personal boundaries that need to be respected, and it's important to understand and accept your partner's limits. If a woman doesn't want to talk about a certain topic or doesn't feel comfortable in certain situations, it's important to respect her choices and not try to force her to do something she doesn't want to do.

Finally, it's also important to respect a woman's online privacy. In today's digital world, it's crucial to be aware that the information shared online can easily be accessible to anyone, and it's important to respect her privacy by avoiding sharing personal information about her without her consent.

Respecting her space and privacy needs is a sign of respect and maturity that can make a difference in building a healthy and lasting relationship. Showing your partner that you understand her needs and are willing to respect them is a way to demonstrate your love and care for her.

Furthermore, respecting a woman's privacy can help strengthen mutual trust within the relationship. Knowing that you can trust your partner and that your space and privacy will be respected allows you to feel more secure and protected within the relationship.

Ultimately, respecting her space and privacy needs is a fundamental aspect of winning and maintaining a healthy and happy relationship. Showing sensitivity and attention to your partner's privacy can make a difference and help build a deeper and more lasting bond.

23.Strive to Resolve Problems and Conflicts with Maturity

Strive to Resolve Problems and Conflicts with Maturity: The Ultimate Guide to Winning a Woman's Heart

Relationships can be complex and full of challenges, but facing them with wisdom and maturity can help solidify a lasting bond with the person we love. In this article, we will explore some effective strategies for handling conflicts wisely and winning a woman's heart.

Communication is Key

Communication is the foundation of every healthy and lasting relationship. When it comes to resolving problems with a woman, it is essential to communicate openly and honestly. Avoiding or hiding your feelings will only worsen the situation. Instead, it is important to address issues head-on and speak sincerely. Listen carefully to the woman's perspective and try to understand her needs and concerns. Effective communication is fundamental for resolving problems and building a stable and lasting relationship.

Show Empathy and Understanding

When facing a problem with a woman, it is crucial to show empathy and understanding. Putting yourself in her shoes and trying to understand her emotions and motivations can help create a more harmonious and favorable environment for resolving the conflict. Showing empathy towards her will demonstrate that you genuinely care about her feelings and are willing to work together to find a solution. Empathy and understanding are essential qualities for building a healthy and lasting relationship.

Maintain Calm and Patience

When dealing with a conflict with a woman, it is vital to maintain calm and patience. Anger and frustration can further complicate the situation and escalate it into a fight. Instead, it is important to stay calm and try to resolve the problem in a serene and rational manner. Keeping calm during a discussion can help control emotions and find a peaceful and constructive solution. Patience is a precious virtue when it comes to resolving problems with a woman and can help overcome difficulties with wisdom and maturity.

Be Willing to Compromise

In relationships, conflicts and differences of opinion are inevitable. When facing a conflict with a woman, it is important to be willing to compromise. Giving up part of your pride or beliefs to find common ground can help resolve the conflict effectively and maintain peace within the relationship. Being flexible and open to compromise will show her that you are willing to set aside your ego for the sake of the relationship, which can strengthen the bond between the two partners.

Try to Learn from Conflicts

Conflicts and disputes are an integral part of every relationship and can offer valuable opportunities for personal growth and learning. When facing a problem with a woman, it is important to try to learn from the experiences and use conflicts as an occasion to improve yourself and your relationship. Reflecting on your actions and the dynamics of the relationship can help identify recurring issues and develop effective strategies for dealing with them in the future. Using conflicts as opportunities for personal and relational growth can lead to greater self-awareness and a healthier, more satisfying relationship.

Facing problems and conflicts with maturity is essential to winning a woman's heart and building a strong and lasting relationship. Communicating openly and honestly, showing empathy and understanding, maintaining calm and patience, being willing to compromise, and learning from conflicts are all effective strategies for handling conflicts wisely and constructively. By following these guidelines, it will be possible to face the challenges of a relationship with wisdom and maturity, creating a deep and lasting bond with the loved one.

24. How to Win Over a Woman and Capture Her Attention

Winning over a woman may seem like an insurmountable challenge for many men, but there are actually some simple tips that can help you capture her attention and win her heart. In today's article, I'll provide some suggestions on how to attract a woman and make your approach more effective.

First of all, it's important to understand that every woman is unique and has her own preferences, so there is no magical formula that works for everyone. However, there are some general guidelines that can help you maximize your chances of success.

The first step in winning over a woman is to show genuine interest in her. Listen attentively when she speaks and ask questions about her life, interests, and passions. Showing that you are sincerely interested in getting to know her will help you create a deeper and more meaningful connection.

Additionally, it's important to be authentic and genuine when approaching a woman. Don't try to be someone you're not; instead, show your true self and be honest about your intentions. Women appreciate sincerity and transparency, so try to be yourself and present yourself authentically.

Another important tip is to show confidence in yourself. Women are attracted to men who are self-assured and know what they want. Maintain good posture, make eye contact, and speak with determination. Self-confidence is an irresistible attraction for many women, so work on yourself and develop a sense of security.

Furthermore, it's important to show respect and kindness toward the woman you're interested in. Behave with courtesy, kindness, and respect, and treat her with the same consideration you wish to receive. Women are attracted to kind and thoughtful men, so strive to be a true gentleman when you're with her.

Another useful suggestion is to be fun and engaging. Women appreciate humor and lightheartedness, so try to be funny and positive when you're with her. Tell jokes, make her smile and laugh, and try to create a light and pleasant atmosphere. A man who can make a woman laugh is definitely an attractive man!

Finally, it's important to be patient and not rush things. Building a meaningful and lasting relationship takes time and effort, so try to be patient and give the relationship time to develop naturally. Don't be too anxious or pushy, but let things take their course and allow the connection between you to grow slowly but steadily.

Winning over a woman and capturing her attention requires effort, sincerity, and authenticity. Show genuine interest, self-confidence, respect, and kindness, and you will be well on your way to winning the heart of the woman you desire. Follow the tips provided in this article and you will surely be able to achieve success in your love life. Good luck!

25.Useful tips to conquer a woman:

1. Speak to her with respect and kindness

2. Show interest in what she says and does

3. Give her sincere compliments

4. Smile often and look into her eyes

5. Listen attentively when she speaks

6. Make her feel special to you

7. Always be honest with her

8. Surprise her with small gestures to make her feel loved

9. Dedicate time to get to know her better

10. Make her feel safe and protected by your side

11. Show your affectionate and caring side

12. Be there for her in difficult times

13. Respect her opinions and feelings

14. Be open and available to communicate

15. Solve problems together instead of avoiding them

16. Make her feel proud of herself

17. Support her in her goals and passions

18. Create romantic and special moments for her

19. Be a good listener

20. Support her in achieving her dreams

21. Show your fun and cheerful side

22. Let her know she is your priority

23. Respect her space and time

24. Be present in her daily life

25. Surprise her with romantic and caring gestures

26. Remember her preferences and passions

27. Always pay attention to what she likes and dislikes

28. Bring her back down to earth to show her she is important

29. Dedicate time to your relationship

30. Plan romantic trips together

31. Make her feel heard and understood

32. Accept and respect her opinions

33. Show your sensitive side

34. Treat the people important to her with respect too

35. Show gratitude for the things she does for you

36. Be affectionate and caring

37. Always smile when you are with her

38. Make her feel like she can rely on you

39. Let her know you are there for her at any time

40. Plan special moments for just the two of you

41. Express your feelings clearly and honestly

42. Let her know you are proud of her and her achievements

43. Make her feel desired and loved

44. Dedicate time to care for your relationship

45. Show her you are willing to commit to her

46. Give thoughtful and meaningful gifts

47. Plan romantic dinners and special evenings

48. Keep the passion and desire alive

49. Show your tender and sensitive side

50. Let her know you are by her side at all times.

Index